Eating Paleo For Beginners

Pros and Cons of Eating Paleo

By: Bring On Fitness

© Copyright 2019 – Bring On Fitness – All Rights Reserved.

By reading this document, the reader agrees that under no circumstances is the author responsible for any losses, direct or indirect, which are incurred as a result of the use of information contained within this document, including, but not limited to, errors, omissions, or inaccuracies.

About Bring On Fitness

Our passion for fitness gave life to **Bring On Fitness**. We started with the goal of helping as many people as we can. To educate, motivate and to help change peoples lives for the better. Bring On Fitness is not only for the fitness enthusiasts, but also for the beginner. We strongly believe nothing is more important than learning the basics and creating a strong foundation in both nutrition - through meal planning, and in exercise - by following a specific plan. This is just as important for the beginner, as it is for the experienced athlete.

We set high standards for ourselves, the information we share, and the products we carry. Our goal is to provide you with exceptional products that suit your needs and the knowledge and motivation to help you work towards and achieve your health and fitness goals.

Keep up to date by liking us on Facebook and Instagram @bringonfitness

For more check us out at:

https://www.northstarreaders.com/bringonfitness

"Our Mission is to have a positive impact in changing peoples lives. We will deliver the best possible fitness and nutrition solutions that will empower people to achieve their health and fitness goals."

Table of Contents

Introduction

I want to thank you for purchasing the book, *"Eating Paleo For Beginners: Pros and Cons of Eating Paleo."*

When you decide to change your lifestyle or follow a diet, the first thing you must do is understand the benefits and risks associated with the same. You may have a heard a great deal about the benefits of eating Paleo and how it aids in weight loss. However, it is best to understand if this diet is meant for you and if it is easy for you to follow this diet. Adapting to a Paleo will require you to change the types of food you currently consume and also the ways that you prepare it.

This book will give you information on Paleo and help you understand the benefits of this diet. You will also learn information on the types of food you must include and those that you must avoid when you follow eat following the Paleo method. You will learn to focus on eating right and stop counting the calories that you consume. Before you adapt to a new lifestyle or change your diet, you must understand whether the diet will work for you. This book will help you understand if Paleo is indeed the right diet for you.

Thank you for purchasing the book. I hope you obtain all the information you are looking for.

Chapter One: What is Paleo?

The word *"Paleo"* is derived from *"Paleolithic,"* which is the era of our ancestors. Paleo is about following the path of our ancestors and eating just like they did. Most people are obese and are prone to developing obesity-related disorders because they lead a sedentary life and rarely eat healthy. People have only now realized the importance of following a healthy diet. Paleo gained fame because it comprises only of foods that were hunted and gathered in the Paleolithic era.

Paleo followers believe that our digestive systems have not undergone much change since caveman days. Most parts of the Paleolithic era were before agriculture began. These people believe that food like legumes, potatoes, salt, cereal grains, dairy, refined sugar, root vegetables, processed foods, and refined vegetable oils put a strain on our digestive system.

If you compare the physique of Homo sapiens then and now, you will notice that the human beings in the Paleolithic era were agile, muscular, incredibly versatile, and athletic, whereas now, most human beings are out of shape, overweight, unhappy, stressed out, sleep deprived, and dying from diseases because of bad lifestyle choices. There are some people who will have you believe that Paleo is not good to follow because cavemen did not survive very long. This is not an argument that one needs to dwell on because it is important to understand that medical advancements have increased the lifespan of every human being in this era. If the same medical treatments were available in the Paleolithic era, we might have met some of our forefathers.

What do you think changed? Most people believe that lifestyles began to change when human beings discovered farming a few thousand years ago. Humans went on to become farmers rather than hunter-gatherers, and they settled in groups that led to civilization as it is today. Each group of individuals adopted a lifestyle that adhered to the type of food they began to cultivate. Human beings began to consume more grains and sugar because those were the easiest crops to cultivate. Unfortunately, our bodies are unable to adjust to this change.

There is no right way to eat. Even Paleolithic humans followed a variety of diets that were dependent on what food was available to them. Some ate a high-carb diet with quite a lot of plants while others ate a low-carb diet that comprised mainly of animal foods. Eating Paleo is based on the following principles:

- **Consume unprocessed and wholesome food** – the kind that is rich in nutrients and will provide your body with a whole lot of energy. The food groups that are included in this category are fruit, vegetables, meat, eggs, nuts, and seafood. Always be mindful of purchasing unprocessed varieties. This will do away with the possibility of chemicals entering your system.
- **Avoid the types of food that will affect your metabolic process**es like large quantities of gluten, sugar, salt, and artificial food.

Chapter Two: What to Eat and What to Avoid

Before you make the effort to understand the science behind Paleo, you must first identify the types of food you can eat and the food you must avoid. Some people may find it challenging to keep up with this diet just because they cannot think about variety and repeat the same foods every day. This need not be the case; Paleo will push you into coming out of your comfort zone and exploring other food categories that you would have normally not thought of.

Here are some foods to choose from if you want to give paleo a try. You will need to fuel your body with a lot of natural and unprocessed foods and fats, including the following options:

What to Eat

There are some people who are under the impression that Paleo is all about the consumption of meat because, in their mind, the hunter-gatherers only ate meat. However, if they spent some time on research, they would understand that human beings in the Paleolithic era ate all types of food that were available to them. You must only remember to stick to whole and unprocessed food.

- Eggs (preferably free range)
- Nuts and Seeds
- Fish and other seafood
- Fresh seasonal fruit
- Non-starchy vegetables
- Healthy oils like coconut, walnut, olive, flaxseed, avocado, and macadamia (in moderation)

Fruit and Vegetables

Fruit and vegetables are abundant in fiber, antioxidants, vitamins, and minerals. You can consume every fruit and vegetable you can find, but ensure that you eat these in moderation. There are some vegetables, like potato, that are starchy and some fruit like bananas, which contain sugar. You must ensure that you understand the nutritional content of every fruit and vegetable you consume to ensure that you meet your goals.

Eggs

Eggs are rich in Vitamin B, antioxidants, protein, and minerals. Eggs are easy to prepare and are affordable. It is best to buy cage-free or organic eggs because they are rich in Omega-3 fat.

Nuts, Seeds, and Healthy Oils

Nuts and seeds are rich in fiber, protein, and healthy fats. Both nuts and seeds were foraged in the Paleolithic era. Therefore, you can load up on them.

The oils listed in the section above are allowed because they are extracted directly from plants. You may wonder why flaxseed oil has been included in the list above because hunter-gatherers probably never consumed it. However, this oil is allowed because it is rich in Omega-3 fatty acid and alpha-linoleic acid (ALA), which is an anti-inflammatory fatty acid that also promotes heart health.

What to Avoid

Eating Paleo is all about eating clean and real food. As mentioned earlier, this diet is not very rigid. However, there are quite a few food groups that you must avoid. This chapter will walk you through those foods, the ones that you may have been eating for a quite some time, or ones you find tasty or even consider to be healthy!

There are different versions of Paleo, but in most cases, the following foods are to be avoided:

- Refined Sugars
- All types of dairy products (including milk, yoghurt, cheese, and butter)
- Legumes (like peas, beans, and peanuts)
- Fruit juices and soft drinks

- Cereal grains (like rice, wheat, rye, and barley)
- Excess salt
- Sweets (including candy, sugar, and honey)
- Cured and processed meats (like hotdogs, bacon, and deli meats)
- All processed foods

Gluten

Gluten is a mix of proteins that are found in many of the foods that we consume. Commonly found in rye, wheat, and barley, this is one compound that is known to cause digestive problems in the majority of the population. These digestive problems lead to hormonal imbalances because the immune and endocrine systems are responsible for healing the body.

Grains

Human beings have been consuming grains since they began to farm. You may be surprised that this food group has made it to this list. Grains contain many compounds, such as lectins, gluten, and phytic acid, which have adverse effects on the human body. Additionally, grains are rich in carbohydrates. When you consume more carbohydrates, your body will never burn fat because it has a sufficient amount of carbohydrates that can be used to produce energy.

Seeds and Nuts

You may wonder why this category has made its way into both lists. Seeds and nuts contain many molecules of lectins and phytic acid. These will be covered in brief in the next sections of this chapter. However, you can consume the nuts and seeds that have been mentioned in the earlier section. Additionally, you can soak every nut and seed you in water before you consume them. When you soak them, you remove some of the lectins and phytic acid, thereby rendering those nuts and seeds harmless.

Lectins

This compound is present in most food that is consumed and is also found in the human body. These are proteins that protect living beings against all kinds of diseases. Wheat Germ Agglutinin, commonly known as WGA, is a type of lectin found in most grains, beans, nuts, and seeds. This lectin latches onto the inner surface of the small intestine and tricks your body into accepting it as a necessary substance. When your body identifies that these substances are causing harm to your body, antibodies are generated. These antibodies do not attack the lectins but attack the organs because lectins have the ability to function like any organ in the human body, which leads to the development of autoimmune diseases.

Phytic Acid

Phytic acid is one of the many acids that cannot be broken down in the human body because the enzyme required to digest it, phytase, is not produced by the body. This acid is found in most grains and nuts, and its molecules latch onto minerals like magnesium, calcium, zinc, and iron in any part of the body, thereby preventing their assimilation. Human beings often develop deficiency diseases because of phytic acid.

Legumes

Legumes or beans are not as harmful as grains. However, they contain gluten and other harmful substances. This means that you must reduce your intake of legumes. It is best to soak them overnight and then cook them fully before you consume them. It is also best to consume legumes when they are fermented and well sprouted because this reduces the phytic acid and lectins. Artificially manufactured legumes through genetic modifications are very harmful to the body. They affect the immune system and also increase gas in the body.

Refined Sugar

Refined sugar is a sweeter variant of normal sugar and is made up of simple carbs. This sugar is made from corn, beets, and sugar cane. Some chemical alterations are made to these items before they are processed to extract refined sugar

When you consume large quantities of sugar, your blood sugar increases, making the blood toxic to your body. This increase in blood sugar levels leads your body into believing that it needs to release insulin to convert the glucose in your blood to glycogen. Given that so much sugar is consumed, the body does not have the ability or the capacity to produce more insulin to convert glucose into energy. Therefore, the sugar remains in your blood, and some of the converted glucose is stored in the body as fat.

When you consume more sugar, you will be tired and sluggish and will want to consume an energy drink or caffeine. These products release the adrenaline and cortisol hormones. The latter is known to release some stored glucose into the bloodstream to produce energy, whereas the former is known to revive your system. These hormones give your body the impression that it has been in a near death experience. If this happens continuously, you may develop many health issues.

Two serious issues that one may develop as a result of this vicious cycle are:

- **Type II Diabetes**: When your body begins to produce more insulin to break the glucose molecules down, it will become resistant to insulin. The cells in your body will begin to absorb insulin instead of using the smaller glucose molecules to produce energy. This increases blood sugar levels, leading to diabetes.
- **Your body may secrete cortisol continuously**. This hormone can control the endocrine system and can shut the immune system down, leading to multiple disorders and organ failures.

Vegetable Oils

Most vegetable oils are not extracted from vegetables and are most certainly not healthy for your body. These oils are extracted from the seeds of the plant. These oils contain large quantities of fat. When this fat enters the human body, it is oxidized and broken down into soluble and insoluble fats. These insoluble fat molecules move to the bloodstream and accumulate at different parts of the body, leading to inflammation.

Chapter Three: Pros and Cons of Eating Paleo

Now that we have covered the basics of eating Paleo, let us take a quick look at the pros and cons of the diet. You can make an informed decision about the diet once you fully understand the content of this chapter.

Benefits associated with the Eating Paleo

Muscle Gain

Eating Paleo likely means you will be eating foods rich in protein, which is an essential nutrient that aids in the formation and repair of muscles and tissues. If you visit the gym regularly, you must follow this diet because you will consume protein that will help you grow lean muscles. You can stay fit and healthy when you follow Paleo because the food consumed in this diet not only strengthens your muscles but also helps to maintain some fat around the muscle.

Weight Loss

When you shift to eating Paleo, you begin to consume whole and unprocessed food. These food types are known to keep your hunger satiated for a long period because these foods are rich in fiber. When you follow Paleo, you must avoid the consumption of aerated drinks, chips, cookies, butter, some oils, and sweets. When you remove these food types from your diet, you will begin to lose weight because you will reduce your caloric intake. When you burn more calories than you consume, you will begin to lose weight.

Increased Fertility

Leptin is a protein that has a direct effect on the central nervous system. This protein controls your food intake, cravings, and reproduction. When you follow Paleo, you will consume foods that are rich in leptin. If you want to reap the benefits of leptin, you must avoid grains and legumes because they decrease the leptin found in your body.

Good Sleep

Serotonin and melatonin are two hormones that help to regulate the sleep cycle. These hormones are found in abundance in seafood and meat. When you consume more of these foods, you can ensure that you have a good night's sleep. Serotonin is a hormone that is also known to keep a person happy.

Better Digestion

When you follow Paleo, you consume foods that are rich in fiber. Fiber is a component that is known to aid in digestion and also provide relief to those suffering from digestive disorders, such as constipation and irritable bowel syndrome.

Better Libido

When you drop the unwanted weight and also get a good night's sleep, you begin to feel better about yourself. You will have more energy, which helps to increase your libido. You will also become more confident about yourself because your hormones will finally strike a balance.

Clear Skin

When you remove all the junk, oil, and sugar from your diet, your face will begin to clear out. Given that you consume less oil, your sebaceous glands will not produce too much sebum or inflammation to cause acne and pimples on your face. Given that your body is clean from the inside, your skin will glow.

Risks and downsides associated with Eating Paleo

- When you follow Paleo, you are expected to remove some food groups from your diet. This may mean that you are reducing your intake of nutrients present in such food. For example, when you remove dairy from your diet, you are reducing your intake of calcium and Vitamin D. Experts suggest that this reduction may lead to osteoporosis, fractures, and rickets.
- As mentioned earlier, some people believe that Paleo is a meat-centric diet. If you consume too much meat, you may develop cardiovascular diseases because the concentration of the LDL cholesterol will increase in your body.
- When you avoid carbohydrates for a long period, your body will shift into a metabolic state called ketosis where fat reserves are used to produce energy, which can be harmful for some people.
- It is difficult to commit to a diet that removes multiple food groups. When you lose weight on this diet, you may be unable to sustain that weight loss because you cannot always be consistent on a diet. There may be times when you may have to switch to a normal diet for a few days, weeks, or maybe even months.
- This diet can be quite difficult for vegetarians to follow as it restricts the consumption of beans and grains, which are important components of their diet.
- This diet can get heavy on the pockets because you must always consume fresh and wholesome food. This means that you will shell out more money to purchase healthy food, such as organic vegetables, grass fed beef, free-range chicken, and eggs.

- There is not enough scientific evidence to justify the many benefits of eating Paleo. It is harder to understand whether the diet is beneficial in the long run. Most studies are not significant statistically, and there are no clinical studies to back those statistics.
- It is important to consult a physician if you have any medical conditions. If you plan to switch from eating Paleo to a low-carb diet while following Paleo, you must consult your physician to ensure that there are no consequences.
- It becomes difficult to enjoy a meal outside with your friends and family because you follow a strict diet.

Who will Benefit from the Eating Paleo

Like other diets, eating Paleo also has some food groups that you must avoid or reduce in quantity. It can be difficult for some people to stick to Paleo and most other diets because they are restricting some foods they are used to consuming. That being said, it is important to understand whether Paleo is indeed beneficial to you. This chapter sheds some light on who should follow and who should avoid eating Paleo.

Those who would benefit

As mentioned earlier, eating Paleo helps to manage Type II diabetes, and there is some research being conducted to fully justify this claim. A recent study was conducted on two groups of people to understand how Paleo changes blood sugar levels. One group was asked to follow Paleo for two weeks, while the other was on a normal diet that included the consumption of legumes, grains, and dairy. After two weeks, the blood sugar levels were measured, and the group following Paleo had stable blood sugar levels. More studies must be conducted to better understand the benefits of eating Paleo. This diet is also beneficial to those who are on their weight loss journey.

Those who should avoid

As mentioned earlier, eating Paleo is beneficial to those suffering from Type II diabetes. That being said, it is important to consult your doctor and understand how this diet affects your blood sugar levels and if it is good for you. It is dangerous for a person suffering from Type II diabetes to have a steep dip in his or her carbohydrate intake. You must consult your doctor and understand if you need to change your medication when you are on this diet.

If osteoporosis runs in your family, you must consult a doctor before you start this diet because there is some debate on the intake of Vitamin D and calcium. If you do choose to start on this diet, you must monitor your intake of these nutrients. If you suffer from health conditions, such as kidney disease or cardiovascular diseases, check with your physician before you begin this diet.

Chapter Four: Tips to Help You on your Paleo Journey

Now that you understand what eating Paleo is and have decided on whether or not the diet is for you, let us take a look at some tips that will make your journey easier.

- Most households have different types of junk food, such as chocolates, chips, aerated drinks, fruit juices, and other processed food, which they must never consume when on the Paleo. The first step would be to remove this junk. It may be difficult to get rid of these foods because we often call them "comfort food" and consume packets of this food when we have bad days. However, you must throw all these packets into the trash without giving it a second thought.
- In the earlier chapters of the book, you have gathered information on the food groups that you must avoid. Try to remove any food from your pantry that falls into those groups. Your body must be given time to adapt to change, so instead of giving up on these food groups all at once, get rid of one group at a time.
- Many are unable to differentiate between good and bad carbohydrates and fats. This means that people often fail to conduct research before they begin a new diet. You may have come across some people who are following Paleo because they are just following the crowd. It takes some time to understand the nuances of the diet, but you should ensure that you do take these points into account.

- Keep some snacks ready. You may wonder what types of snacks are allowed on this diet, as most items you consider snacks have already been removed from your pantry. However, there are different types of snacks that adhere to the rules Paleo. If you are unsure of what snack to eat, check out some Paleo forums.
- You must make a conscious effort to avoid the junk section in the supermarket. Make a list of the products you need to buy, and put only those items in your cart. If you do happen to pick a product that is not on your grocery list, ask yourself twice if you truly need that product.
- When you officially begin eating Paleo, your body will begin to detox. This is a difficult stage for most people because their cravings start to kick in. Stay strong, and munch on some Paleo friendly snacks if you need to consume some food to help you get over the cravings.
- Always plan your diet out. When you start a new diet, it gets tricky if you do not plan because you do not know what meals to prepare for lunch or dinner. You may then succumb to your old habits and eat a sandwich or some junk. To avoid this, plan your days in advance, and try to prepare all your meals for the week and then stock them in your refrigerator.
- If you live in a large family, ensure that everybody is made aware about your choice to change your diet. You can include some or all members of your family on your journey.
- Always focus on the results. Try to avoid being negative, and do not worry about what you are giving up on.
- Give yourself the freedom of cheat days. Cheat days help most people stick to their diet with renewed focus.

Once your body is used to eating clean, you will stop craving junk.

- You must change the way you think. Most people are afraid of diets because they are worried about what they will miss out on. Stop calling it a diet, and focus on the benefits you will reap from making a change in your lifestyle. Always believe that what you are doing now will help you lead a healthy life.

- It is hard to stick to a new diet or adapt to a new lifestyle. However, it will get easier. If you are tempted to eat more junk or miss your favorite cookies, give yourself a reward on your cheat day. Alternatively, you can take up an activity that makes you happy. When you perform activities you are passionate about, your brain will release the hormone oxytocin, which will communicate to your body that you are happy.

Conclusion

Thank you for purchasing this book.

Obesity and its health-related disorders have increased over the last decade. Most people understand that they must change their lifestyle and their eating habits to ensure that they lead a healthy life. Many nutritionists, cardiologists, and scientists have developed multiple diets that people can adopt to shed all the extra fat from their body. Eating Paleo is one such diet. However, this diet, unlike the other diets, does not cost too much. All you must do is switch to the diet of your ancestors.

I hope that you are convinced that eating Paleo is for you. It is hard to shift from a relaxed lifestyle to a strict lifestyle quickly. There are many things you must bear in mind, and there are times when this may overwhelm you. To make this transition easier for you, this book has left you with some tips that you can use during the first few days or weeks into the change. Remember to include wholesome meals and only consume real food. Try to include more vegetables and fruit into your diet.

Thank you for purchasing the book. I wish you luck on your journey.

Thank you, and remember to share how well these Paleo Diet Tips work for you. You can do that by writing a review in your Amazon account under Your Orders.

Thank you,

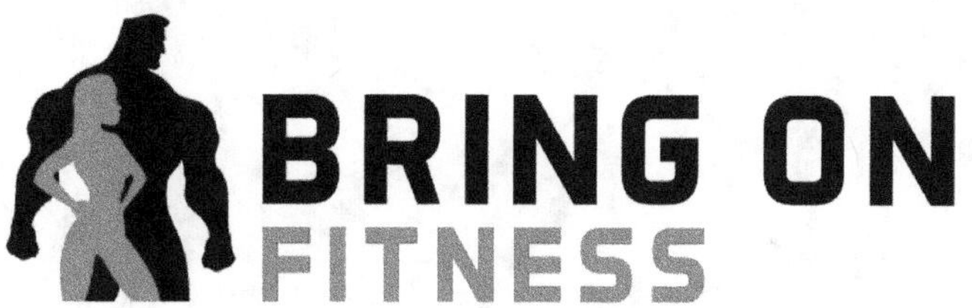

9 781707 468980